Jesus is Lord
Addiction is Not

A self-study course on
overcoming addiction

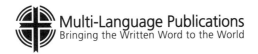

Multi-Language Publications
Bringing the Written Word to the World

Original text produced by the Institutional Ministries
Committee of the Commission on Special Ministries of the
Wisconsin Evangelical Lutheran Synod

Copyright © 2000

Text adapted by Multi-Language Publications of the
Wisconsin Evangelical Lutheran Synod

Printed in 2002
Second Printing - 2010

ISBN 1-931891-02-8

Book 10

Table of Contents

Getting Started

This book will help you learn some exciting things about Jesus Christ, your Savior. Each chapter begins with a list of goals marked with a small star (*). These goals tell you what you will be learning in that chapter. Then you will read a few lines and answer some questions. At the end of the chapter there is a test. The test questions cover only what you read in the chapter and the questions you have completed.

When you finish answering a group of questions, you will be given a page number where you can turn to check your answers. If you turn to that page, you will find the answers at the very bottom of that page. Check your answers carefully, correcting any mistakes you made. Make sure you understand all the answers before reading any further.

At the end of the chapter there is also a section marked Using Your Bible. There you will be told where in the Bible you can find the stories talked about in the lesson. If you are able, try to read the stories directly from your own Bible. We want you to be sure that what this course is teaching is exactly what the Bible teaches.

At the end of the book there is a final test. Before you complete the test, go back and review the chapter tests. When you complete the final test, you can either turn it in to the person who gave you this book, or mail it to the address on the back cover.

May God help you to learn more about Jesus Christ, and bless the hours you spend studying his life.

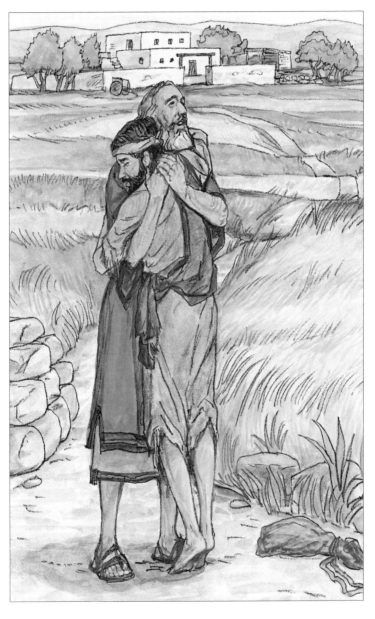

*The father hugged his son, forgave him,
and welcomed him home.*

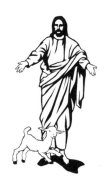

Chapter One

IT IS GOING TO TAKE SOMEONE GREATER THAN YOURSELF TO FREE YOU

An addict is someone who is mentally and physically dependent on something like alcohol or drugs. When an addict is cut off from his drug, he does not think, "It would be kind of fun to get high [under the effects of drugs] again." His body and mind are screaming, "You have to get high again! You need your drug!"

It is not just people who get high that have an addiction problem. Jesus said, "Everyone who sins is a slave of sin" (John 8:34). Things like hatred or pride or lust or worry will hook you just as surely as crack cocaine [a drug]. When you use sin to try to meet your needs, you are not really using sin; sin is using you.

God does not want anybody to be a slave of an addiction. The Bible has much to say about God's plan and his power to free you from addiction's slavery. Jesus said, "If the Son of Man [Jesus] sets you free, you will really be free" (John 8:36). In this book you are going to get a look at some of what the Bible says about getting free of the power of addictions. We are going to use twelve steps of recovery from alcohol as an outline for this study.

Here are the 12 Steps:

1. We admit we are powerless over alcohol -- that our lives have become unmanageable.

2. Come to believe that a power greater than ourselves can restore us to sanity.

3. Make a decision to turn our will and our lives over to the care of God, as we understand him.

4. Make a searching and fearless moral inventory of ourselves.

5. Admit to God, to ourselves, and to another human being the exact nature of our wrongs.

6. Be entirely ready to have God remove all these defects of character.

7. Humbly ask him to remove our shortcomings.

8. Make a list of all persons we have harmed and become willing to make amends to them all.

9. Make direct amends to such people wherever possible, except when to do so would injure them or others.

10. Continue to take personal inventory, and when we are wrong promptly admit it.

11. Seek through prayer and meditation to improve our conscious contact with God, as we understand him, praying only for knowledge of his will for us and the power to carry that out.

12. Having had a spiritual awakening as the result of these steps, we try to carry this message to alcoholics, and to practice these principles in all our affairs.

Reprinted with permission - AA World Services, Inc.
Twelve Steps and Twelve Traditions

In this chapter you are going to look at:

* how addictions take over a person's mind and life so powerfully; and

* why it is going to take God's almighty power to set you free.

If you get a cut and you do not clean it up a

dangerous infection might enter your body through that cut. Addictions are like a spiritual infection. Just like an infection in your body, they can enter you through a wound. Maybe your parents hurt you or left you when you were little. Maybe you have tried very hard to get people to like you, and you failed. Things like that wound a person's spirit. And if you start getting high, the addiction gets into you through those wounds.

Drugs take away the pain of being ashamed or lonely or angry for a little while. Then you find yourself wanting to get high more and more often so you never have to feel that pain any more. The infection gets worse, and you spend more and more of your time and money on getting high. You start doing things like lying, hurting, or stealing from the people you love. The Bible says, "I will not be controlled by anything" (1 Corinthians 6:12). But that is exactly what happens to someone who becomes addicted. The task of getting high takes over your life.

1. Addictions are like a spiritual

_____.

2. Things like abuse or feelings of failure give you a wounded _____, and addictions can enter you through those wounds.

3. Getting high keeps you from feeling _____, and the task of getting high takes over your _____.

(Check your answers on the bottom of page 10)

One reason cravings for drugs can take over so powerfully is because there is a spiritual force behind the addiction. Think of how liquor stores advertise that they sell "Wine and Spirits." The Bible says a lot about evil spirits, called demons, taking over people's lives and torturing them. Those same evil spirits get at people through drugs, take over their lives and torment them.

Satan has lots of ways to trap you -- drugs and

alcohol, sex outside of marriage, or hate and pride and worry. As a result, you are powerless to get yourself out of that trap. You might have told yourself and the people who cared about you, "I can quit any time I want to." But that is a lie. In the Bible the apostle Paul wrote, "I know there is nothing good in my sinful nature. I want to do what is good, but I can't. I don't do the good things I want to do. I keep on doing the evil things I don't want to do. I do what I don't want to do. But I am not really the one who is doing it. It is sin living in me…The sinful mind is at war with God. It does not obey God's law. It can't. Those who are controlled by their sinful nature can't please God" (Romans 7:18-20, 8:7-8).

That is why the First Step says, "We admit we are powerless over alcohol, that our lives have become unmanageable." You do not have the power to fight your way out of the trap the devil has laid for you.

4. Drugs take over an addict so powerfully because evil _____ can use them to take over people's lives.

5. The power of sin living in you can keep you from doing the _____ you want to do and make you do the _____ you do not want to do.

(Check your answers on the bottom of page 12)

But God is not powerless. God's power is greater than any other power, including the evil powers behind addictions. The Bible says God chose to love you and set you free from the devil's trap through his Son, Jesus. Jesus left heaven and came into our world. He was born as a human being. He took all the blame for what we have done wrong off of us and put it all on himself. That is what happened when Jesus died on the cross. When you put your trust in Jesus you have complete forgiveness for everything you have ever done, said or

---

? Answers for page 8: 1. infection; 2. spirit; 3. pain, life.

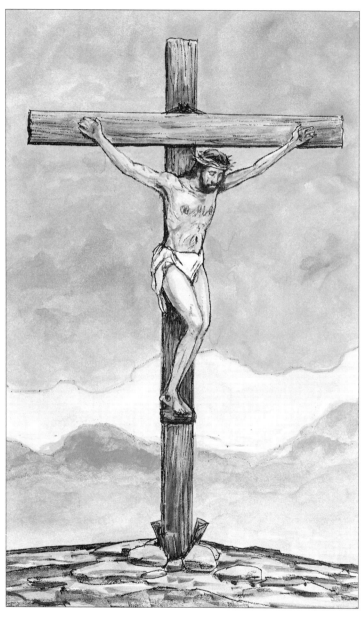

Jesus suffered and died for the sins of all people.

thought that was wrong. The Bible says, "Give glory and power to the One who loves us! He has set us free from our sins by pouring out his blood for us" (Revelation 1:5). That means when you trust in Jesus as your Savior, you can be sure of going to heaven when you die.

But you might be thinking, "That is great, but I am not dead yet. Right now my addiction is pulling me into sin and away from the life God wants for me. Can God do anything about that?" The answer is yes. The Bible says, "The Son of God came to destroy the devil's work" (1 John 3:8). What Jesus did by dying on the cross includes destroying the devil's trap of addiction.

The Second Step says, "We come to believe that a power greater than ourselves can restore us to sanity." The Bible tells us Jesus is that power.

?   Answers for page 10: 4. spirits; 5. good, evil.

6. God's power is _____
than the power of addiction.

7. God sent _____ into our
world to free us from the devil's trap.

8. Jesus took the blame for our _____
on himself and died on a _____.

9. When you trust in Jesus you can be sure of
going to _____ when you die.

10. The power of Jesus can _____
the works of Satan, and restore us to

_____.

(Check your answers on the bottom of page 14)

Review of Chapter One

You have had some bad things happen to you.
These bad things have hurt your spirit. You
have tried to use actions that went against
God's will to ease the pain of those wounds.
You may have used things like drugs, alcohol,

sex outside of marriage, and other things. You may have gotten relief from your pain for a little while. But you got something you had not planned on. You also got an evil spiritual force that started taking over your life and turning you into something you did not want to be. Then you were powerless to free yourself from the control of this evil force.

But God loves you, and he has the power to set you free from the powers of hell trying to keep you down. He showed that love by sending his son, Jesus, who died to take away the blame for everything you have done, said or thought that was wrong. Besides promising to forgive you for your sins and giving you eternal life in heaven, God has promised you power to live a sane life, free from the control of addiction.

?   Answers for page 13: 6. greater; 7. Jesus; 8. sins, cross; 9. heaven; 10. destroy, sanity.

Thought questions:

A) If you do not get high, or when you could not get any drugs, what sinful things have you used to block out the pain of your wounded spirit? (For example: controlling other people, becoming very angry with someone, homosexual activity, spending most of your waking hours doing nothing or working too long and too hard)

B) How have other people tried to tell you they are seeing your life become out of control? What did you tell them (and tell yourself) to try to convince them you did not have a problem?

C) If Jesus is the power greater than yourself, who will restore you to sanity? In what ways does he need to be greater than you are? (For example: able to forgive you when you cannot forgive yourself, able to give you the desire to change your life when you are not even sure you want to try to change)

Test on Chapter One

1. Your spirit has been _____
by bad things that have happened in your life.
The spiritual infection called addiction entered
into your spirit when you _____ _____
to block out the pain in your spirit.

2. You can get temporary relief from your
spiritual pain through drugs, but you can also
get something else along with drugs. An evil
_____ can take control of your
_____.

3. To be honest, you have to admit that you are
_____ over alcohol or
whatever the devil has used to take over your
life.

4. God's power is _____
than the power of addictions.

5. When Jesus died on the cross, he won
_____ for our sins.

6. When you trust in Jesus, you can:

a) hope you are going to heaven.

b) be pretty sure you are going to heaven.

c) be totally sure you are going to heaven.

(Circle the best answer)

7. Jesus has the power to:

a) free you from the control of addiction.

b) help you cut back on your sinning.

c) take you to heaven, but you are on your own in this world.

(Circle the best answer)

(Check your answers on page 73)

Using Your Bible

To find out more about the addictive power of sin, and the greater power of God, you can read the following words in the Bible:

The insanity of addiction: Proverbs 23:29-35

Demons trying to take over people's spirits, and Jesus setting them free: Luke 8:26-39, Mark 9:14-29

Our powerlessness to help ourselves: Romans 7:7-25

God's power to forgive us and set us free from the control of sin: Romans Chapter 8

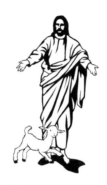

Chapter Two

DO NOT TRY HARDER; SURRENDER

In this chapter we are going to look at what the Bible says about how:

* your new life is a gift from God, not something you work to earn;

* you have a new life because God comes to live in you;

* you have a new life because God gives you a new self; and

* a Christian can let God take charge of his life instead of sin.

You might have had people say they have become full of religion. You know what that is. Someone starts going to church and Bible study and saying, "I used to be a sinner, but praise Jesus! I have seen the light!" Such a person is trying hard to do religious things and say religious words, but has anything really changed inside that person where it counts.

It hurts when people will not believe you have really changed. But maybe such people have their reasons. Maybe there were times when you told people, "I swear this will never happen again! I am changing my ways! This time I really mean it!" And you really did mean it. But still you ended up picking up the bottle of whisky, or the drug pipe, or the gun again. So maybe now nobody trusts you. Maybe you do not know if you can trust yourself, either.

Recovery from addiction does not come from trying hard to take control of your life. You have tried that. Do not waste your time trying harder. Recovery, like salvation, is a gift from God. The Bible has some strong words for all of us who keep trying hard to earn something that we can only receive as a gift. In Galatians 3:1-5 God says, "You foolish people of Galatia! Who has put you under an evil spell? When I preached, I clearly showed you that Jesus Christ had been nailed to the cross. I would like to learn just one thing from you. Did you receive the Holy Spirit by obeying the law? Or did you receive the Spirit by believing what you heard? Are you so foolish? You began with the Holy Spirit. Are you now trying to complete God's work in you by your own strength? Have you suffered so much for nothing? Why does God give you his Spirit? Why does he work miracles among you? Is it because you do what the law says? Or is it because you believe what you have heard?"

God is calling all of us to quit trying to get everlasting life in heaven or to get a new life here on earth by our own works. Just receive God's gift of life in Jesus. That new life includes freedom from the control of addiction.

1. People who try hard to do religious things and say religious words cannot change themselves _____ where it counts.

2. Everlasting life in heaven is something Jesus _____ to give us, and we receive it as a free _____.

3. New life here on earth is also something we receive as a free _____ from Jesus.

(Check your answers on the bottom of page 24)

The Bible says that when God gives you faith in Jesus he does not just give you faith. He gives you himself. In 1 Corinthians 12:3 God says, "Without the help of the Holy Spirit no one can say, 'Jesus is Lord.'" In John 15:4-5 Jesus says, "Remain joined to me, and I will

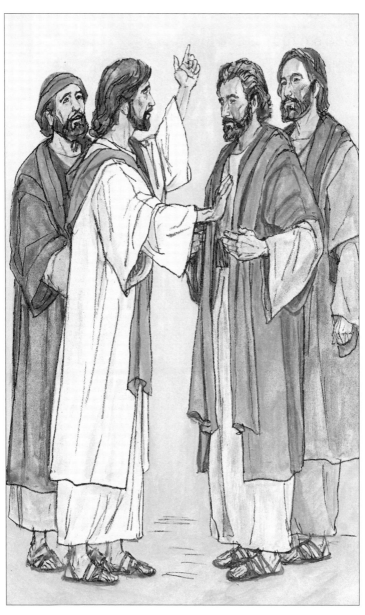

Jesus promised to send the Holy Spirit to his friends.

remain joined to you. No branch can bear fruit by itself. It must remain joined to the vine. In the same way, you can't bear fruit unless you remain joined to me. 'I am the vine. You are the branches. If anyone remains joined to me, and I to him, he will bear a lot of fruit. You can't do anything without me.'"

The Almighty God, the Father, Son and Holy Spirit, has come to live in everyone who trusts in Jesus as his or her Savior.

Living a new life as a Christian does not mean trying hard to help yourself and get your sin under control.

Living a new life as a Christian means getting a new self from God, a new self with Jesus living in you. In Galatians 2:19-20 the apostle Paul says this about his new life in Jesus, "Because of the law, I died as far as the law is concerned. I died so that I might live for God. I

? Answers for page 22: 1. inside; 2. died, gift; 3. gift.

have been crucified with Christ. I don't live any longer. Christ lives in me. My faith in the Son of God helps me to live my life in my body. He loved me. He gave himself for me."

God invites you to believe that he forgives all of your sins. At the same time he invites you to believe he is giving you a new self. God promises he will live in you and be the power for your new life. Your new life includes power over the control of addiction.

4. When God gives you faith in Jesus he also gives you _____ to live in you.

5. Jesus said, "I am the vine. You are the branches. If anyone remains _____ to me and I to him, he will bear a lot of fruit."

6. In Galatians 2:19-20 Paul says, "I have been _____ with Christ. I don't live any longer. Christ _____ in me."

7. God invites you to believe he has given you forgiveness for your sins, and that he is giving you a new _____.

(Check your answers on the bottom of page 28)

Everyone is born a sinner. People who do not have faith in Jesus are stuck with their old sinful selves. They really do not have any choice but to do what their sinful nature tells them to do. When God gives you faith in Jesus, he gives you a new self. That does not mean the old sinful part of you is gone. You still find yourself sometimes thinking sinful things and wanting sinful things. But now sin is not in charge. Now you have the power, through Jesus, to make some real choices. Here are some examples of what the Bible says about the choices Jesus' followers can make, "Brothers and sisters, we have a duty. Our duty is not to live under the control of our sinful nature. If you live under the control of your sinful nature, you will die. But by the power of the Holy Spirit you can put to death the sins your body commits" (Romans 8:12-13).

"Brothers and sisters, God has shown you his mercy. So I am asking you to offer up your bodies to him while you are still alive. Your bodies are a holy sacrifice that is pleasing to God" (Romans 12:1).

"Put to death anything that belongs to your earthly nature. Get rid of your sexual sins and unclean acts. Don't let your feelings get out of control. Remove from your life all evil longings. Stop always wanting more and more…. That's the way you lived at one time in your life. But now here are the kinds of things you must get rid of. You must put away anger, rage, hate and lies. Let no dirty words come out of your mouths. Don't lie to each other. You have gotten rid of your old way of life and its habits. You have started living a new life. It is being made new so that what you know has the Creator's likeness" (Colossians 3:5-10).

"Don't fill yourself up with wine. Getting drunk will lead to wild living. Instead, be filled with the Holy Spirit" (Ephesians 5:18).

If you trust in Jesus as your Savior, you can start living and thinking as the new person God has made you. You can let God be in charge, stopping the remains of your old self from taking over. That is what Christians do when they follow the Third Step: "We make a decision to turn our will and our lives over to the care of God as we understand him."

Think of it this way: suppose for years you shared a room with a very powerful, very negative, and very mean person. He frightens you and steals from you. He has the walls covered with his dirty pictures. He controls what is said so you always end up talking about committing crimes and using drugs. You have to laugh at all his dirty jokes. If he is in a bad mood, he makes sure you are in a bad mood, too. Living with such a roommate is like living in hell because of this person.

Then one day your roommate leaves. You get
a new roommate. He smiles warmly and
shakes your hand, and says, "Hi. I am Jesus."

Now you are sharing your room with Jesus.
What will happen now? Your old roommate left
behind his dirty pictures and his ugly way of
thinking. Are you going to tell your new
roommate, "Let us just leave things the way
they are." Are you going to tell him, "Do what
you want with your part of the room, but leave
my part alone." Are you going to tell him, "I
promise I will try hard to make this room a
nicer place." Or are you going to tell him, "This
is your room now. Do whatever you want with
it, and I will help you. "That is what has
happened to everyone who has come to faith
in Jesus. The person you used to be is gone,
and Jesus has come to live in your heart. But
your old self left an ugly mess behind,
including such things as hatred, lust, cursing
and swearing. Are you going to allow sin to go
on the way it always used to, and say, "That is
just the way I am." Are you going to try to let

Jesus have just some of your life while you keep some other parts to yourself? Are you going to try hard to solve your problems yourself? Or are you going to listen to God's invitation and let Jesus have it all?

8. People who do not have faith in Jesus have no choice but to do what their

_____ _____ tells

them to do.

9. A person with faith in Jesus is:
a) the same person he always was.
b) a better person than he used to be.
c) a new person, with God living in him.
(Circle the best answer)

10. If you believe in Jesus as your Savior, you can now choose to let God be in charge of

_____ _____.

11. If you believe in Jesus as your Savior, you can now choose to:
a) sin less than you used to.

b) no longer let sin be in charge of your life.

c) just accept your sinfulness as part of who you are.

(Circle the best answer)

(Check your answers on the bottom of page 32)

Review of Chapter Two

A person can try to change his life, but if he does not have faith in Jesus from God, or if he is trying to change his life by himself, his efforts are not going to amount to much. He cannot really change himself inside, where it counts. But when God gives you faith in Jesus, he comes to live in your heart and makes you a new person.

Even though a Christian's old person is gone, it left a sinful mess behind, That mess includes things like hatred, lust, cursing and swearing. But the new person God gives you can now say, "Sin is not going to be in charge of my life. Jesus, you take over."

Thought questions:

A) Are there parts of your life you thought you had to be in charge of because you thought it was not God's job? Are there parts of your life that you do not want God to take charge of?

B) What happens when you hold back a part of your life from Jesus?

C) The Bible says you are a new person if you have Jesus as your Savior. But you may feel like the same old person you always were. Are you going to believe what your feelings tell you? Or are you going to believe what the Bible tells you?

Test on Chapter Two

1. Jesus won everlasting life in heaven for us by dying on the cross. We now receive Jesus' salvation as a free _____.

2. A new life (including a life free of the control of addictions) is also something we receive as a free _____.

3. You were born with a sinful _____.

4. In Galatians 2:19-20 Paul writes, "I have been _____ with Christ. I don't live any longer. Christ _____ _____
_____."

5. God invites you to believe that he has given you forgiveness for your sins, and that he is giving you a new _____.

6. Since God has made every Christian into a new person with Jesus in his heart, every Christian can choose to let Jesus be in charge of _____

_____.

(Check your answers on page 73)

Using Your Bible

To find out more about God's gift of a new self
or person, a new life and power over sin, read
about it in the Bible:

The sinfulness everyone is born with: Psalm
51:1-5, Romans 8:3-9

The Christian's new self or person, united with
Jesus: John 15:1-8, Romans 6:1-4, Colossians
3:1-4, Ephesians 2:1 -10

The Christian's power to let Jesus be in
charge, instead of sin: Romans 6:5-14, 8:1-17,
Titus 2:11-14

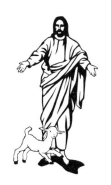

Chapter Three

HOUSECLEANING

Tony was starting to live a Christian life. He had given up using drugs. After a few months he decided to go to his mother's house for Christmas. While he was there the police showed up. In times past Tony had broken the law. Tony had some old charges out on him that he had never taken care of. He had forgotten about them, but the police did not. And now Tony was put in jail.

Anybody who has started to live the new life that Jesus gives is like Tony. Even though you are born again, you bring some problems along with you from your old life. Such problems may be the ways you hurt other people and the ways other people hurt you. Just like Tony's old problems, those problems from your old life can get you into real trouble if you do not do something about them.

In this chapter we are going to look at what the Bible says about how:

*   the devil tries to get at you through sins and shames of the past; and

*   repentance is God's way of getting the devil's control out of your life.

Have you ever started out your day with good intentions, or hoping to do good? You say, "Lord God, my life is in your hands. I am going to live today as your child." Then before you knew it you have became angry with somebody or did some other sin? It made you wonder or think, "What is wrong with me?" That is exactly what you need to find out.

The Fourth Step says, "We make a searching and fearless moral inventory of ourselves." The Eleventh Step says, "We continue to take personal inventory and when we are wrong promptly admit it." The Bible talks about doing the same thing. For example, in Psalm 139:23-24 the Bible says, "God, see what is in my heart. Know what is there. Put me to the test. Know what I'm thinking. See if there is anything in my life you do not like. Help me live in the way that is always right."

1. Is having good intentions enough to make sure you live right and avoid sin? _____

2. To find out what is getting in the way of living right you need to take a "searching and fearless _____

_____."

3. In Psalm 139 the Bible says to pray that God
will _____ your mind and
_____ you live in the way that is
always right.

(Check your answers on the bottom of page 40)

You can say, "Jesus is Lord of my life," and
mean it. But there still may be parts of your life
that you are keeping Jesus out of, and you do
not even know it. That is why you need to let
God shine his light into your mind and life and
see what the devil is using to get at you.

Get to know the Bible, first of all, so you can
understand what God is like. Learn what he
wants and does not want. Then the Holy Spirit
can help you:

*   get in the habit of regularly reading the
     Bible and praying on your own;

*   get together with other Christians for Bible
     study and prayer sessions; and

*   go to worship services and find out about the Bible from church leaders.

The Eleventh Step says, " . . . seek through prayer and meditation to improve our conscious contact with God as we understand him, praying only for knowledge of his will for us and the power to carry that out." You need to have the truth about God to meditate on, if your meditation is going to be any good. That is why you need to get to know God's true message to people, the Bible. As you get to know God's truth, you can start to write down the truth about yourself, your moral inventory. You need to list what you have discovered about yourself, both good and bad. This will help you see where God has already made changes in you and where more changes are needed. It will help you see if there are any parts of your life where you are holding back from God and trying to run your own life. It will help you see what parts of your life the devil may be using to try to turn you away from God and back to getting high.

Take your time. Ask for help from other people you trust. Be honest. Nobody ever has to read what you are writing but yourself, so you do not need to impress anyone. Pray that God will show you what he wants you to know about yourself. Trust that when Jesus died on the cross he paid for all the sins you find when you examine yourself. You will not find anything God has not forgiven.

4. How are you going to know what God is like, what he wants and does not want?

_____

_____

5. Three ways you can get to know the Bible better are:

1)

2)

3)

? Answers for pages 37-38: 1. No; 2. moral inventory; 3. know, help.

6. Writing down your moral inventory will help you see where God has made _____ in you, what parts of your life you are _____ _____ from God, and what parts of your life the devil may be using to try to _____.

(Check your answers on the bottom of page 42)

Then what? Step Five says, "We admit to God, to ourselves, and to another human being the exact nature of our wrongs." That is also what the Bible tells us. For example, in James 5:15-16 God says: "If you have sinned, you will be forgiven. So admit to one another that you have sinned. Pray for one another so that you might be healed."

There is a saying, "You are only as sick as your sickest or worst secret." If you have been carrying a secret shame around for a while, it could be making you do things and say things you really do not want to do or say. It could be giving the devil a way to get at you. The Bible calls the devil the accuser. He tries to bring up your secret shames and make you think, "I am a loser. I might as well give up." You can mess up the devil's plans by admitting what is wrong in your life to someone you trust, especially if that person is a Christian who can talk to you about God's love and forgiveness. (A pastor or minister can be helpful because keeping things he hears a secret is part of his job.)

7. The Bible calls the devil the _____ because he tries to bring up your secret shames and make you feel like you are hopeless.

8. When you admit what is wrong to another Christian, that Christian can talk to you about God's _____ and

_____.

(Check your answers on the bottom of page 44)

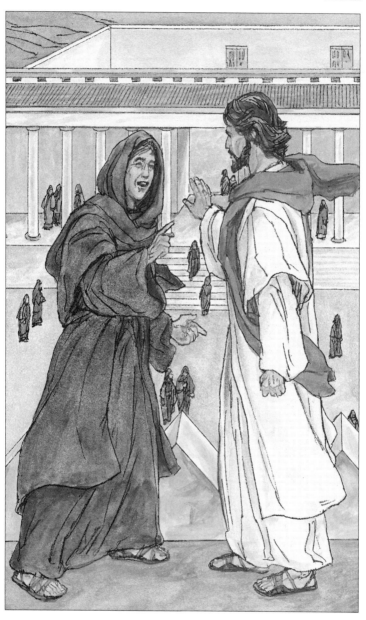

Jesus told the devil that he would not sin against God.

Now if you were still thinking in your old way, you would probably be saying something like, "Now that I have found out what is wrong with me, I just have to work hard to make myself a better person." Think back to the First Step where you admit you are powerless over your sins, and to the Second Step where you come to believe that only a power greater than yourself, God, can and will restore you to sanity.

Do not ever believe the lie that God just tells you what is wrong with yourself, and then leaves it up to you to fix what is wrong. God never says, "Now it is up to you." Instead of thinking it is all up to you to change yourself, you need to think and to pray the thought spoken of in Psalm 51, "Wash me. Then I will be whiter than snow. Let me hear you say, 'Your sins are forgiven.' …God, create a pure heart in me. Give me a new spirit that is faithful to you…Give me a spirit that obeys you. That will keep me going."

That is why, instead of talking about how you should work hard being a better person by yourself, Steps Six and Seven say, "We are entirely ready to have God remove all these defects of character," and "We humbly ask him to remove our shortcomings."

God wants you to leave behind your old way of thinking and living and have a new mind, a new heart and a new life. The Bible calls this repentance. You do not produce this repentance yourself. Like every other good thing in life, you receive it as a gift from your loving God. "My dear brothers and sisters, don't let anyone fool you. Every good and perfect gift is from God. It comes down from the Father. He created the heavenly lights" (James 1:16-17).

"God's grace has saved you because of [through] your faith in Christ. Your salvation doesn't come from anything you do. It is God's gift. It is not based on anything you have done. No one can brag about earning it. God made us. He created us to belong to Christ Jesus. Now we can do good things. Long ago God prepared them for us to do" (Ephesians 2:8-10).

[Jesus says,] "Everyone the Father gives me will come to me ... No one can come to me unless the Father who sent me brings him" (John 6:37, 44).

9. It would be wrong to think that, once you have found out what is wrong with you, that it is up to you to _____ _____ ____ _____.

10. God's gift of a changed mind, heart and life is what the Bible calls _____.

(Check your answers on the bottom of page 48)

You have probably made many promises to many people that you would change your ways. You have probably broken a lot of these promises. Maybe you thought the problem you were trying to change was simple and you would be able to just try hard and the problem would go away. Now maybe you are ready to come to God and admit, "I cannot figure out what is wrong with me! I want to change but I just cannot find the way to do it! Will you please show me what is wrong, and will you please make it right"? God will not turn down such a prayer!

Review of Chapter Three

When you start your new life with God, you bring along many things from your old life. You bring along things like memories of hurt and shame and sinful habits of thinking and living. You may not even be aware of all that old baggage, but it is real and it can get in the way of your new life with God. You need to know God's Word, the Bible. Then you can understand what God is like and see where your thinking and living are different from God's ways. You need to take a moral inventory of yourself. You need to list what you have discovered about yourself, both good and bad. The bad things need to be admitted to God, to yourself and to another person you can trust. The best choice would be another Christian who can assure you that Jesus died to give you forgiveness for what is wrong. Then pray to God to change what is wrong, and trust that he will be patient and loving and work with you to change what is wrong.

Thought questions:

A) There is a saying among those who are recovering from alcoholism that says, "My problem is 10% alcohol and 90% me. Why do you think they say that?

B) How have secret shames gotten you to do things that were wrong? (Examples: a man who was sexually molested as a child may have sex with as many women as he can just to prove to himself that he is really a man. A woman who aborted her baby may go out and get drunk every year on the anniversary of the abortion.)

C) Have you, or people who know you well, seen changes in yourself since you started trusting Jesus, even though you had not really tried to make those changes?

Test on Chapter Three

1. Sin and shame from a person's past are:
a) no problems for a Christian.
b) something the devil can use to get to a Christian.
c) something Christians should try to just forget.

(Circle the best answer)

2. An honest look at what is wrong and what is right with you is called:

a) a moral inventory.

b) making amends.

c) self-improvement.

(Circle the best answer)

3. If you are going to know what God wants and does not want for you, the book you have to get to know is _____ _____.

4. You need to admit the truth about what is wrong with you to _____, to _____, and to another _____   _____.

5. When you admit your sins to another Christian, he can assure you of Jesus' _____.

6. Leaving behind your old way of thinking and living and receiving a new way of living and thinking from God is called:

a) repentance.

b) tithing.

c) confirmation.

(Circle the best answer)

(Check your answers on page 73)

Using Your Bible

To find out more about what the Bible says about working with God to search yourself, and to receive God's gift of repentance, read:

Psalm 51

Luke 5:1-11

Luke 18:9-14

Acts 9:1-21

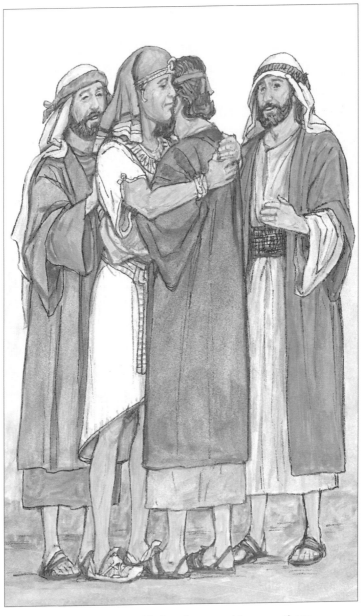

Joseph hugged his brothers and forgave them.

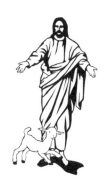

Chapter Four

JESUS CHANGES THE WAY YOU RELATE TO PEOPLE

Jesus changed your relationship with God. He took away your guilt and paid for your sin with his blood and brought you into God's love. Jesus changed your relationship with yourself. You do not have to lie to yourself or hate yourself anymore because now you are a holy and loved child of God. Jesus also changes your relationship with other people.

Maybe you have used people to get what you wanted. Maybe you hurt a lot of people that way. Maybe you have been hurt by other people, and you have been carrying that hurt around for years. It has made you into a mean, angry person who does not trust anyone. But now Jesus is in your life, and the Bible says, "From now on we don't look at anyone the way the world does. At one time we looked at Christ in that way. But we don't anymore. Anyone who believes in Christ is a new creation. The old is gone! The new has come!" (2 Corinthians 5:16-17).

In this chapter you are going to look at what the Bible says about:

*   making amends to people you have sinned against; and

*   sharing what God has given you with other people.

Perhaps in your life you hurt someone very badly. You may have had the person you hurt testify, in court, about how you hurt them and their family. As you listened to them tell about how much pain you brought into their lives, maybe you wished you could do something to make up for the bad you did.

The great news is you do not have to do anything to make up for the hurt you have caused. You could not help even if you wanted to. Jesus took over your guilt when he went to the cross. He paid for your sins in full when he died. God is completely satisfied with the payment Jesus made for your sin. You can be completely satisfied, too.

But there may still be some people out in the world who are not satisfied. They may still be hurting because of wrongs you have done against them. These may include not only victims of crime but your own family and friends. They may be people you let down, people who have broken hearts and lives because of what you have done. God wants to heal their hurts. He wants you to be part of that healing wherever and whenever you can.

Steps Eight and Nine say:

8. Make a list of all persons we harmed and become willing to make amends to them all.

9. Make direct amends to such people wherever possible, except when to do so would injure them or others.

Jesus says the same thing in Matthew 5:23-24, "Suppose you are offering your gift at the altar. And you remember that your brother has something against you. Leave your gift in front of the altar. First go and make peace with your brother. Then come back and offer your gift."

Pray for God's help. Then start looking at ways you can make amends to people. This might include:

*   apologizing (in person or by letter);

*   paying back what you have stolen or destroyed;

*   taking the blame for sins you have been denying up till now.

Making amends is not easy. It will probably be hard to do. But you will be working with Jesus as he works to heal those people's hurts. You will gain a new closeness with Jesus that will be greater in value than the problems it will cost you.

1. Jesus' death on the cross _____ _____ all the wrong you have done.

2. God is completely _____ with the payment Jesus made for your sins.

3. If there are people who are still hurting from the wrongs you have done to them, you need to make _____ to them.

(Check your answers on the bottom of page 58)

There are other hurting people in the world, too. They are hurting because they do not have Jesus in their lives. They are trying to use other things to put happiness and peace in their lives. Such things may be drugs and alcohol. They do not love Jesus, but he loves them. Jesus wants them to have new life with him just as he has given new life to you. Jesus said in John 10:14-16, "I am the good shepherd ... I give my life for the sheep. I have other sheep that do not belong to this sheep pen. I must bring them in too. They also will listen to my voice. Then there will be one flock and one shepherd."

The Twelfth Step says, "Having had a spiritual awakening as the result of these steps, we try to carry this message to alcoholics and to practice these principles in all our affairs." The one thing that can set alcoholics and all other sinners free is trusting Jesus.

| ? | Answers for page 57: 1. paid for; 2. satisfied; 3. amends. |

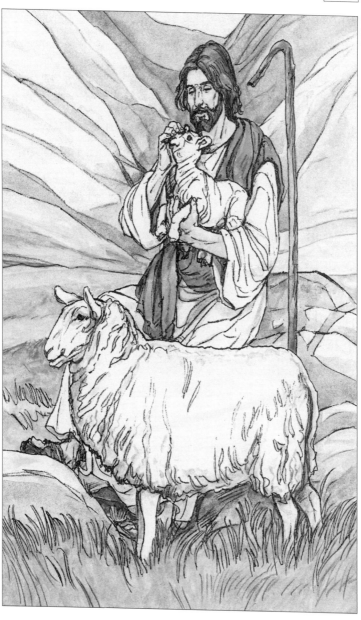

Jesus is our Good Shepherd.

You cannot force anybody to trust in Jesus. That is not his way of doing things. His way is to invite people to trust him. That is where we come in.

Some ways you can introduce people to Jesus are:

*   talking to them about who Jesus is and what a difference he has made in your life;

*   giving them Bibles and good Christian books; and

*   inviting them to Bible studies and to worship services.

Maybe you are not used to talking with people about personal things like your faith. Maybe you are used to keeping to yourself. Maybe you are nervous about people rejecting you if you talk about Jesus with them. That is all right. Admit it to Jesus. Pray for him to do something about it. Watch as he makes a way for you to talk about him with people who are ready to listen. Watch the Holy Spirit make your new family, the family of believers, grow.

4. The one thing that can set alcoholics, addicts and other sinners free is

_____ _____.

5. Jesus calls people into his family by:
a) commanding them.
b) threatening them.
c) inviting them.
(Circle the best answer)

6. Three things you can do to introduce people to Jesus are:
A.
B.
C.
(Check your answers on the bottom of page 62)

A pastor was leading a Bible study a few years ago. Most of the men in the study happened to be black or Hispanic. A person who was white came in late and gladly joined the class. He was grateful to be able to study God's Word together with other believers. When the study was done and it was time to pray, the white person happily joined hands in prayer with the black and Hispanic people. After the Bible study the white man stayed behind to thank the pastor for leading the study. That is when the pastor noticed the tattoos on the inmate's arms that included swastikas, racist slogans, and neo-Nazi gang symbols. The man noticed the pastor looking at his arms, and he explained, "That was all from a different life. I am with Jesus now." Jesus had brought this man from a narrow little family of hateful racists into a big loving family of all believers. Jesus wants still more people to come into his family. Pray to him to make you part of the process!

Review of Chapter Four

When Jesus comes into your life and brings you salvation, your relationship with other people changes. You start to love them and to care about their pain. If their pain has been caused by something you have done, you work on making amends to them. If they are hurting because they do not have Jesus in their lives, you pray to God to bring them into God's family. You let God lead you in introducing them to Jesus and inviting them to trust him as their Savior.

Thought Questions:

A) Sometimes people set out to apologize to the ones they have hurt. They speak in a way that excuses what they did, or makes it seem like it is not important. Or they even blame the ones who were hurt for causing the problem. What kind of apology does God want you to make?

B) How does it help you in making amends to know that God already forgives you before you make your amends?

C) Maybe the person you need to apologize to will not forgive you. Why is it still important to apologize?

D) What are some things you can do if you talk to someone about Jesus and he rejects what you are saying?

Test on Chapter Four

1. You do not make up for the wrong you have done; Jesus made up for it by _____

_____ _____ _____.

2. Making amends to the people you have hurt does not earn you forgiveness from God, but it can help:

a) heal the hurt those people have suffered.

b) make those people like you again.

c) impress people.

(Circle the best answer)

3. Making amends might mean apologizing to the people you have hurt; it might also mean

_____   _____ what you have stolen or destroyed, or taking the

_____ for sins you have been denying up until now.

4. People turn to drugs and alcohol mainly because:

a) they are not happy with life.

b) all their friends are getting high.

c) they are missing a relationship of trust with Jesus.

(Circle the best answer)

5. Arguing about religion is not Jesus' way of reaching out to people. His way is to

_____ people to get to know him and trust him.

6. Telling people about Jesus and what he has done for you is one way to reach out to people who are hurting. You can also give them _____and invite them to come to _____ _____ and _____.

(Check your answers on page 73)

Using Your Bible

Making amends:

Luke 19:1-10

Ephesians 4:21-5:21

Introducing people to Jesus:

Luke 8:26-39, especially verses 38-39

Acts 17:19-34

1 Peter 3:15-16

Colossians 4:2-6

Glossary

(A list of words you may not know)

abort to end before the expected time

abortion the act of ending the life of a baby before it is born naturally

accuser one who says you have done wrong

advertise to make known something is for sale

alcoholic a person who must drink wine, beer or other such liquids

addict a person who must have alcohol or drugs

addiction a continuing need for something

amends to make right the wrongs you have done to people

apologize to say you are sorry for a fault or for causing pain

ashamed feeling shame, guilt or sorrow

baggage things to carry

bandage a strip of cloth used to cover a wound or injury

character here it means a special quality in someone

choice the act of selecting something

commit to do something wrong

compassion pity for someone who is in need or suffering

conscious on purpose, deliberate

convince to cause someone to believe what is said is true

corrupt totally sinful

crave a deep desire to have something

crime an act that is against the law

crucifixion being nailed to a cross to die

decision a conclusion, a choice or judgment

defect something not perfect; a fault

deny to refuse to accept what is true

dependent to happen because of something else

exact correct, accurate

examine to question or to look at

exciting	to have strong, pleasant feelings of happiness
fix	to make right
habit	what you do again and again
high	in this book to be under the influence of drugs
Hispanic	someone of Spanish origin
homosexual	attracted to a person of the same sex
honest	full of truth
hook	make you depend on or need something
impress	to cause someone to respect you
improve	to make something better
infection	a disease from germs that get into a cut or bruise
injure	to hurt
intention	what you plan or want to do
inventory	a listing of facts about ourselves
liquor	a strong alcoholic drink
meditation	thinking about God and his ways

memories things you think about that happened in the past

mess trouble; disorder; confusion

message words spoken or written

miracle wonderful act done with God's help

molest to attack sexually

mood the state of a person's feelings

moral having to do with right or wrong in our character

obscene dirty and filthy

pen where sheep are kept safe at night

perversion turning something good into something wicked (for example, love into lust)

principles general truths, rules or laws

promptly right away, immediately

quit to stop

racist a person who believes people of one color are better than people of another color

recovery the act of getting back what was lost

reject not wanting to be your friend or accept what you say

relate to have a relationship

relationship a connection with other people or with God

relief help

religion belief and worship of a god

repentance turning away from sin to faith in Jesus and to a godly life

restore to bring back to what something was before

sacrifices offerings to God

salvation being saved from going to hell

sanity the ability to live in the real world and not do something crazy; soundness of mind

satisfy to please someone by meeting his needs

scream a loud shouting noise

secret something known to you and kept from others

self person

shame an act that brings dishonor

slogan a statement of the aim of a person or group

solve to find an answer to a problem

spirits another word for liquor or other alcoholic drink

spiritual nature your Christian nature, the part of you that wants to obey God's laws

swastika a sign or symbol

tattoo a permanent mark or design made on the skin

temporary lasting only for a short time

testify to make a statement about the truth of something

thoroughly completely

torment to worry

torture to cause great suffering in a person

trap something to catch and hold something

victim someone who suffers because of what someone else has done

wound a hurt to your body or to your feelings

Answers to the Chapter Tests

Chapter Test One: (Pages 16-17)

1. wounded or hurt, got high; 2. spirit, life; 3. powerless;
4. greater; 5. forgiveness; 6. c; 7. a.

Chapter Test Two: (Pages 32-33)

1. gift; 2. gift; 3. nature; 4. crucified, lives in me; 5. person;
6. his life.

Chapter Test Three: (Pages 49-51)

1. b; 2. a; 3. the Bible; 4. God, yourself, human being;
5. forgiveness; 6. a.

Chapter Test Four: (Pages 64-66)

1. dying on the cross; 2. a; 3. paying for, blame; 4. c; 5. invite;
6. Bibles, Bible study, church.

Final Test

Congratulations! You have completed your study of Jesus is Lord, Addiction is Not. Go back through the book and review any mistakes you made in the chapter tests. Also review the goals from each chapter. When you are confident or sure you know all the goals, you are ready to take the final test.

Complete the final test without looking at the book. When you are finished, give the test to the person who gave you this book or mail it to the address on the back cover. You may also ask for more Bible study books in this series.

If you are ready, remove the test from the book and put the book away. Take the test without opening the book.

Jesus is Lord, Addiction is Not
Final Test

1. An addict keeps getting high because:

a) he feels like it.

b) it is fun.

c) his mind and body tell him he has to.

2. In John 8:34 Jesus said, "Everyone who sins is

a _____ _____

_____."

3. When you use sin to try to get your needs met you really are not using sin; sin is

_____ _____.

Wounded bodies; wounded spirits:
Write **B** in the blank for wounds or hurts that happen to your body. Write **S** in the blanks for wounds or hurts that happen to your spirit.

4. _____ Memories of being abused

5. _____ Resentments

6. _____ Cuts

7. _____ Embarrassment

8. _____ Broken bones

9. _____ Shame

10. _____ Tooth decay

11. _____ Hopelessness

True or false:
Write **+** for true and **0** for false

12. _____ Evil spiritual powers can get into you
when you get high.

13. _____ No sinner can stop doing sinful things by
will power and good intentions.

14. _____ Jesus took care of the guilt of our sins
by dying for them on a cross.

15. _____ You can never be completely sure you
are going to heaven.

16. _____ God does not have the power to free
you from the control of addiction.

17. _____ A new life comes to Christians because they try hard to live right.

18. _____ Freedom from the control of addiction is a gift from God.

19. _____ God is far away in heaven, so it is up to us to make our own lives right.

20. _____ When God put faith in Jesus into your heart, he came to live in your heart.

Circle the best answer:

21. When the Bible says that God gives you a new self, it means:
a) you do not have any sinfulness in you any more.
b) you can now have God be in charge of your life instead of sin.
c) not much has changed, except that you now believe in Jesus.

22. Surrendering your life to Jesus means:
a) trying your best to live right.
b) letting him take over the job of managing your life.
c) going to church all the time.

23. You get to know who God is and what he wants by:

a) getting to know the Bible.

b) looking into your heart.

c) looking at the world around you.

24. As you honestly look at who you are and what you have done, you will find:

a) you are not as bad as you thought.

b) nothing that God does not already know, and nothing Jesus has not forgiven.

c) some things that are too bad to be forgiven.

25. The Bible calls Satan:

a) the evil god.

b) the king of the universe.

c) the accuser.

26. If you admit your sins to a fellow Christian, he can tell you:

a) you are forgiven for everything because Jesus died for you.

b) how to make up for the wrong you have done.

c) that you should be ashamed of yourself.

27. Repentance means:

a) being sorry for your sins.

b) turning your sins over to God for him to forgive and make things right.

c) promising to try hard to live right.

28. You cannot make up for the hurt you have caused other people. _____ did it for you by dying on the cross.

29. If you know someone is hurting because of something you did, you can try to make _____ to that person.

30. If you know people who are hurting because they think they are all alone in this world and it is up to them to fix their own problems, you can invite them to get to know and trust in _____.

Please PRINT the following information.

NAME:_____

ADDRESS:_____

_____

_____

Please give us your comments on this course.

_____

_____

_____

_____

_____

_____

_____

_____

_____

_____

_____